Table of Contents

INTRODUCTION

Your gut is your gastrointestinal system and includes your stomach, intestines and colon. It digests and absorbs nutrients from food and excretes waste.There is no clear definition of gut health, and it can mean something different for researchers, medical professionals and the community. Throughout this page, we refer to gut health as having a healthy gut microbiome and limited digestive symptoms. About 200 different species of bacteria, viruses and fungi live in your large intestine. The bacteria and other micro-organisms in your gut are known as your gut microbiome. The bacteria help to break down food, turning it into nutrients your body can use.

Certain types of bacteria in your gut may contribute to some diseases. Some microorganisms are harmful to our health, but many are beneficial and necessary for a healthy body. We are learning that the variety of bacteria in your gut is an important indicator of the health of your microbiome.The health of your gut can impact both your physical and mental health. Many factors, including the foods you eat, can impact the type of bacteria found in your digestive tract. What we eat can have short-term and long-term effects on our gut microbiome environment.

WHY GUT HEALTH IS IMPORTANT

The gut breaks down the foods you eat and absorbs nutrients that support your body's functions. The importance of the gut to our overall health is a topic of increasing research in the medical community. Research is showing us that our gut microbiome can affect every organ in our body. It is understood that there are links between gut health and:

the immune system

mental health

autoimmune diseases

endocrine disorders – such as type 2 diabetes

gastrointestinal disorders – such as irritable bowel syndrome and inflammatory bowel disease

cardiovascular disease

cancer

sleep

digestion.

A higher level of diversity in gut bacteria is an important indicator of the health of your microbiome. While research is ongoing, it appears that your gut health plays an important role in your overall health.

Signs of an unhealthy gut

Your gut microbiome can be affected by:

stress

too little sleep

lack of physical activity

eating too many ultra-processed foods

smoking and drinking alcohol

taking antibiotics.

The gut microbiome is also affected by things we cannot control, such as our environment, age, birth mode and whether we were breast-fed or bottle-fed as a baby. While we cannot use one specific measure for our gut health, some signs that you may have poor gut health include:

digestive symptoms – such as gas, bloating, constipation, diarrhoea and heartburn

sleep disturbances or fatigue

mood/emotional state – such as high stress, low mood or anxiety

high frequency of infectious illnesses – such as the common cold.

How to improve your gut health

You may be able to improve your gut health through lifestyle and diet changes.

Dietary fibre in foods can improve your gut health as it can help keep us regular, reduce the risk of bowel cancer and feed the healthy bacteria in our gut.

Wholefoods, such as fruits, vegetables, legumes, wholegrains and nuts,

may prevent the growth of some bacteria linked to diseases and inflammation.

Our lifestyle, for example physical activity, good sleep and stress reduction are also good for gut health.

Gut health and diet

Your gut bacteria are influenced by what you eat. It is important to give them the right fuel to have a balanced gut microbiome. The best way to maintain a healthy microbiome is to eat a range of fresh, wholefoods, mainly from plant sources like fruits, vegetables, legumes, beans, nuts and wholegrains.

Eat a high fibre diet

Fibre is important for our gut health for many reasons. Fibre can affect the function of our gut, for example, the digestion and absorption of nutrients, how quickly or slowly things move through and the quality of our stools. The breakdown of fibre by our gut bacteria can also create important products which can influence the development of gastrointestinal conditions such as bowel cancer.

Fibre has other benefits to our health apart from the gut, for example, reducing our risk of developing heart disease and type 2 diabetes.Fibre is only found in foods that come from a plant. Australian adult women should be aiming to eat at least 25g of fibre a day, and men 30g. Foods that are high in fibre include:

vegetables

beans and legumes

fruit

bread and cereals

nuts and seeds.

Prebiotic fibres, which are not found in all high fibre foods, may be especially helpful for our gut microbiome, as they can act as a fertiliser for the healthy bacteria in our gut. They are found in some types of:

vegetables – for example leek, onion and garlic

legumes – for example chickpeas, beans and lentils

wholegrains – for example rye bread, barley and oats

nuts – for example pistachios, cashews and almonds.

Eat a diverse range of food

Eating a wide range of fruits and vegetables ensures you're including a whole range of vitamins, minerals and nutrients in your diet.nThe diversity of food on your plate can help lead to a more diverse microbiome, which is an indicator of a healthy gut microbiome.

Aim to eat at least 30 different types of plant-based foods a week.

Limit ultra-processed foods

Eat foods that are as close to their natural state as possible to support your gut health. While almost all foods have had some kind of processing, it is best to eat foods that are minimally processed. These foods retain their nutritional value and do not usually have added sugar, salt, unhealthy fats or additives such as emulsifiers and artificial sweeteners, all of which may impact your gut health. Unprocessed foods include fruits, vegetables, wholegrains, unflavoured dairy, eggs, seafood, poultry and lean red meat. Ultra-processed foods include deli meats such as ham and salami, many breakfast cereals, ready-made meals, sweet desserts and many packaged snacks such as chips.

Drink water

Water is the best fluid to drink and provides benefits to gut health. Water assists with the breakdown of food, so that your body can absorb nutrients. Water also assists with softening stools, helping prevent constipation. Drinking plenty of water may also be linked to increased diversity of bacteria in the gut.

Eat foods rich in polyphenols

Polyphenols are plant compounds that may beneficially impact our gut microbiome. Foods rich in polyphenols include:

herbs and spices

colourful fruits and vegetables

nuts and seeds

green and black tea

coffee

cocoa and dark chocolate.

Eat slowly

Chewing your food thoroughly and eating slowly may reduce digestive discomfort such as gas, pain and bloating.

Eat fermented foods

Fermented foods have undergone a process in which their sugars are broken down by yeast and bacteria. Fermented foods include:

yoghurt

kimchi

sauerkraut

kefir

kombucha

tempeh.

While research into fermented foods is limited, the bacteria found in some fermented foods have been linked with digestive health and other benefits.

Gut health and probiotic supplements

It is best to improve your gut health through food and other lifestyle factors rather than supplements. There are many nutrients in wholefoods that cannot be packaged into a single supplement. Nutrients in foods also interact with each other in a helpful way and this cannot be replicated in a pill. Many people are interested in taking probiotic supplements. If you're in good health, it is generally not necessary to take a probiotic for your gut health.

In some cases, there is research to support taking a probiotic, however just like medications, you need to take a specific probiotic for the health condition you are trying to manage. Before taking probiotics or any other supplement, it's a good idea to speak to an accredited practising dietitian and your general practitioner to see if it's safe and which one might work.

Gut health and antibiotics
While antibiotics can be very important and useful, they can also have a negative impact on your gut microbiome. Antibiotics aim to kill the harmful bacteria when you have an infection or illness, but in doing so they can remove some of the beneficial bacteria in your gut.

WATER – A VITAL NUTRIENT

The human body can last weeks without food, but only days without water. The body is made up of 50-75% water. Water forms the basis of blood, digestive juices, urine and perspiration, and is contained in lean muscle, fat and bones.bAs the body can't store water, we need fresh supplies every day to make up for losses from the lungs, skin, urine and faeces (poo). The amount we need depends on our body size, metabolism, the weather, the food we eat and our activity levels.

Water in our bodies

Some facts about our internal water supply include:

Body water content is higher in men than in women and falls in both with age.

Most mature adults lose about 2.5 to 3 litres of water per day. Water loss may increase in hot weather and with prolonged exercise.

Elderly people lose about 2 litres per day.

An air traveller can lose approximately 1.5 litres of water during a three-hour flight.

Water loss needs to be replaced.

Importance of water

Water is needed for most body functions, including to:

Maintain the health and integrity of every cell in the body.

Keep the bloodstream liquid enough to flow through blood vessels.

Help eliminate the by-products of the body's metabolism, excess electrolytes (for example, sodium and potassium), and urea, which is a waste product formed through the processing of dietary protein.

Regulate body temperature through sweating.

Moisten mucous membranes (such as those of the lungs and mouth).

Lubricate and cushion joints.

Reduce the risk of urinary tract infections (UTIs), such as cystitis by keeping the bladder clear of bacteria.

Aid digestion and prevent constipation.

Moisturise the skin to maintain its texture and appearance.

Carry nutrients and oxygen to cells.

Serve as a shock absorber inside the eyes, spinal cord and in the amniotic sac surrounding the foetus in pregnancy.

Water in our food

Most foods, even those that look hard and dry, contain water. The body can get about 20% of its total water requirements from solid foods alone. The process of digesting foods also produces a small amount of water as a by-product which can be used by the body. Water sourced this way can provide around 10% of the body's water requirements. The remaining 70% or so of water required by the body must come from fluids (liquids).

Recommended dietary fluid intake

The Australian Dietary Guidelines recommend that we drink plenty of water but how much is enough? The amount of fluid your body needs each day depends on several factors, such as:

your gender

age

how active you are

whether you're pregnant or breastfeeding

lifestyle.

How much fluid to drink each day

Infants 0–6 months*   0.7 litres

Infants 7–12 months# 0.8 litres total (with 0.6 litres as fluids)

Girls and boys 1–3 years	1 litre (about 4 cups)

Girls and boys 4–8 years	1.2 litres (about 5 cups)

Boys 9–13 years	1.6 litres (about 6 cups)

Boys 14–18 years	1.9 litres (about 7–8 cups)

Girls 9–13 years	1.4 litres (about 5–6 cups)

Girls 14–18 years	1.6 litres (about 6 cups)

Men 19 years+	2.6 litres (about 10 cups)

Women 19 years+	2.1 litres (about 8 cups)

Pregnant girls 14–18 years	1.8 litres (about 7 cups)

Pregnant women 19 years+	2.3 litres (about 9 cups)

Lactating girls 14–18 years	2.3 litres (about 9 cups)

Lactating women 19 years+	2.6 litres (about 10 cups)

* from breastmilk or formula

from breastmilk, formula, food, plain water and other beverages

These adequate intakes include all fluids, but it's preferable that the majority of intake is from plain water (except for infants where fluid intake is met by breastmilk or infant formula). Some people may need less fluid than this. For example, people:

Who eat a lot of high-water content foods (such as fruits and vegetables).

In cold environments.

Who are largely sedentary.

Other people might need more fluid than the amount listed and will need to increase their fluid intake if they are:

On a high-protein diet, to help the kidneys process the extra protein.

On a high-fibre diet to help prevent constipation.

Vomiting or have diarrhoea, to replace the extra fluids lost.

Physically active, to replace the extra fluids lost through sweat.

Exposed to warm or hot conditions, to replace the extra fluids lost through sweat.

Although activity levels affect the amount of fluid needed, there are many factors that influence the fluid needs of athletes during training and competition. For example, it is likely that athletes exercising in mild conditions will need less fluid than athletes competing at high intensities in warm conditions.

How to get enough fluid in your diet

If the idea of having to drink lots of cups of water a day doesn't appeal, don't worry – fluids include fresh water and all other liquids (such as milk, coffee, tea, soup, juice and even soft drinks). Fresh water is the best drink because it does not contain energy (kilojoules) and is best for hydrating the body. Water from the tap is also mostly free and generally available wherever you go. However, milk is about 90% water and is an important fluid, especially for children. Just remember to choose full-fat milk for children under 2 years old and low-fat and reduced-fat varieties for everyone else.

Tea can also be an important source of fluid. Tea can help you meet your daily fluid recommendations, and is a source of antioxidants and polyphenols, which appear to protect against heart disease and cancer. If you prefer to get some of your fluids from fruit, aim to eat whole pieces of fresh fruit instead of having fruit juice – you'll still get the delicious fruity juice (fluids) but you'll also benefit from the bonus fibre and nutrients while avoiding the extra sugar found in fruit juice.

Tips for drinking more water

Add a squeeze or slice of lemon or lime, or some strawberries or mint leaves to plain water to add variety.

Keep a bottle or glass of water handy on your desk or in your bag.

Drink some water with each meal and snack.

Add ice cubes made from fresh fruit to a glass of water.

Limit mineral water intake

Commercially bottled mineral water contains salt, which can lead to fluid retention and swelling, and even increased blood pressure in susceptible people. Limit the amount of mineral water or choose low-sodium varieties (less than 30 mg sodium per 100 ml). If you prefer bubbly water, think about getting a home soda water maker so you can just use tap water and make it fresh when needed.

Fluoride in water

An additional benefit of drinking tap (reticulated or mains) water in Victoria is that, in most areas, fluoride is added to the water. Bottled water does not usually have good levels of fluoride. Fluoridation of tap water helps prevent dental decay and is a safe and effective way of providing dental health benefits to everyone.

Avoid sugary and artificially sweetened drinks

The Australian Dietary Guidelines recommend all Australians to limit their intake of drinks containing added sugar. This includes:

sugar-sweetened soft drinks and cordials

fruit drinks

vitamin-style waters

flavoured mineral waters

energy and sports drinks.

Having sugary drinks provides additional energy (kilojoules) to the diet, but no other essential nutrients. There is strong evidence of the association between having sugary dinks and excess weight gain in both children and adults, as well as reduced bone strength and tooth decay. Artificially sweetened drinks add very little energy (kilojoules) to the diet and therefore do not contribute directly to weight gain. However, artificially sweetened drinks still maintain the 'habit' of drinking sweet drinks. They may also lead to decreased bone density (as people may drink less milk) and contribute to tooth decay due to their acidity.

Dehydration

Dehydration occurs when the water content of the body is too low. This is easily fixed by increasing fluid intake.

Symptoms of dehydration

Symptoms of dehydration include:

thirst

headaches

lethargy

mood changes and slow responses

dry nasal passages

dry or cracked lips

dark-coloured urine

weakness

tiredness

confusion and hallucinations.

If dehydration is not corrected by fluid intake, eventually urination stops, the kidneys fail, and the body can't remove toxic waste products. In extreme cases, dehydration may result in death.

Causes of dehydration
There are several factors that can cause dehydration including:

Not drinking enough water.

Increased sweating due to hot weather, humidity, exercise or fever.

Insufficient signalling mechanisms in the elderly – sometimes, older adults do not feel thirsty even though they may be dehydrated.

Increased output of urine due to a hormone deficiency, diabetes, kidney disease or medications.

Diarrhoea or vomiting.

Recovering from burns.

Who is at risk of dehydration?
Anyone can experience dehydration but there are some people who can be more at risk – such as babies, children and the elderly.

Babies and children

Babies and children are susceptible to dehydration, particularly if they are ill. Vomiting, fever and diarrhoea can quickly cause dehydration. Dehydration can be a life-threatening condition in babies and children. If you suspect dehydration, take your baby or child to the nearest hospital emergency department immediately. Some of the symptoms of dehydration in babies and children include:

cold skin

lethargy

dry mouth

blue tinge to the skin (as circulation slows down)

depressed fontanelle in babies (soft spot on top of the skull where the bones are yet to close).

Elderly people

Older people are often at risk of dehydration due to:

changes to kidney function (declines with age)

hormonal changes

not feeling thirsty (body mechanisms that trigger thirst do not work as well as we age)

medication (for example, diuretics and laxatives)

chronic illness

heat stress

limited mobility.

Getting the right balance of fluid intake

Not drinking enough water can increase the risk of kidney stones and, in women, urinary tract infections (UTIs). It can also lower your physical and mental performance, and your salivary gland function, and lead to dehydration. But did you know that it is possible to drink too much water and cause a condition called hyponatraemia (water intoxication)?

Water intoxication (hyponatraemia)

Drinking too much water can damage the body and cause hyponatraemia (water intoxication), although it is pretty rare in the general population. Hyponatraemia occurs when sodium in the blood, which is needed for muscle contraction and sending nerve impulses, drops to a dangerously low level. If large amounts of plain water are consumed in a short period of time, the kidneys cannot get rid of enough fluid through urine and the blood becomes diluted. Hyponatraemia can lead to:

headaches

blurred vision

cramps (and eventually convulsions)

swelling of the brain

coma and possibly death.

For water to reach toxic levels, many litres of water would have to be consumed in a short period of time. Hyponatraemia tends to occur in people with particular diseases or mental illnesses (for example, in some cases of schizophrenia), endurance athletes and in infants who are fed infant formula that is too diluted.

Fluid retention

Many people believe that drinking water causes fluid retention (or oedema). In fact, the opposite is true. Drinking water helps the body rid itself of excess sodium, which results in less fluid retention. The body will retain fluid if there is too little water in the cells. If the body receives enough water on a regular basis, there will be no need for it to hold onto water and this will reduce fluid retention.

GUT HEALTH FOODS - 15 FOODS FOR GOOD GUT HEALTH

Confused about what to eat and what not to eat? With so much information online about healthy eating, it can be tricky to be sure about what health foods are best for a healthy gut. Food should be varied, colourful and high in fibre however, remember that portion sizes should always be in the right proportions for your energy expenditure and should be eaten at regular intervals throughout the day ideally three meals a day.

1. Yoghurt

Live yoghurt is an excellent source of so-called friendly bacteria, also known as probiotics. Look out for sugar-free, full-fat versions and add your own fruit for a tasty breakfast. Yoghurt drinks can contain high numbers of bacteria that are good for the gut, far more than you would find in a normal yoghurt. Do be mindful though as they can have a high sugar content.

2. Kefir

This probiotic yoghurt drink is made by fermenting milk and is packed with good bacteria (which can help to reduce a leaky gut). It originated in the mountainous region between Asia and Europe, as well as Russia and Central Asia. It also makes a great addition to smoothies and soups, or you can use it as a base for salad dressing (add lemon juice and seasoning).

3. Miso

Miso is made from fermented soya beans, plus barley or rice, and contains a range of goodies such as helpful bacteria and enzymes. A savoury paste used in dips, dressings and soup, it can also be used as a marinade for salmon or tofu. It's a staple of Japanese cooking and suitable if you're avoiding dairy. There is uncertainty within the research that the bacteria effectively reach the gut, nevertheless in regions where Miso is a staple fermented food source the population have better gut health and less bowel disease.

4. Sauerkraut

This is finely chopped cabbage that has been fermented. This great source of probiotics, fibre and vitamins is best known as a German dish, but versions exist in Eastern and Central Europe. Choose a product that has not been pickled in vinegar, as that doesn't have the same benefits. It's delicious served with sausages, and can be cheap and easy to make at home.

5. Kimchi

This Korean speciality of fermented vegetables brings the benefits of probiotic bacteria along with vitamins and fibre. Use it as a lively side dish with meat, salad or eggs. It's so popular that Koreans say "kimchi" in the same way that we say "cheese" when they have their photos taken.

6. Sourdough

This is very fashionable at the moment, but there's a good reason for that. Made by fermenting the dough, it's more digestible than regular bread and its energy releases slowly. It makes fantastic toast too.

7. Almonds

These have good probiotic properties, which means they are a treat for your gut bacteria – high in fibre, and full of fatty acids and polyphenols. A handful of almonds makes an excellent snack when you're feeling peckish.

8. Olive oil

Gut bacteria and gut microbes like a diet of fatty acids and polyphenols. These are found in olive oil. Studies have shown that it helps reduce gut inflammation. Use it for salad dressing or drizzle it over cooked vegetables. Some studies have also found olive oil to be beneficial in easing indigestion problems and can also benefit your pancreas through lowering its requirement to produce digestive enzymes.

9. Kombucha

We all know water is crucial for gut health, but what else can you drink? Kombucha is a fermented tea drink thought to have originated in Manchuria that is full of probiotic good bacteria. It has a sharp, vinegary taste and can be used as a refreshing drink on its own or mixed with fruit and spices. It also makes the base for great cocktails.

10. Peas

Gut bacteria need fibre to flourish, so the more fruit and vegetables you consume the better. Peas are full of soluble and insoluble fibre to help keep your system in balance. Add peas to stir-fries, soups or salads.

11. Brussels sprouts

Much more than a festive staple, they contain the kinds of fibre that good bacteria like and sulphur compounds which help combat unhealthy bacteria such as H pylori. Stir-fry with garlic and bacon for a delicious side dish.

12. Bananas

One of nature's handiest and healthiest snacks, bananas are full of the kind of fibre that good bacteria enjoy. They also contain healthy minerals.

13. Roquefort cheese

Live, runny, smelly French cheese* will give your gut bacteria a boost – but eat it in moderation. Add it to salads or spread it on your sourdough. Whilst we cannot be ensured that all of the bacteria survive digestion to be beneficial it is believed that other properties help preserve some bacteria during digestion.

14. Garlic

Garlic, with its antibacterial and antifungal properties, can help keep "bad" gut bacteria under control and help balance yeast in the gut. Use it as a flavouring for savoury dishes. The properties within garlic act as a fuel source to allow the bacteria to do their job better which overall improves gut function and can help heal your gut.

15. Ginger

Fresh ginger can help in the production of stomach acid and it stimulates the digestive system to keep food moving through the gut. Add fresh grated ginger to soups, stews, smoothies or stir-fries. Pour boiling water on grated ginger to make refreshing ginger tea.

Probiotics and prebiotics – what are they and do i need them?

Your intestines host a community of diverse bacteria to make up your gut microbiome. Probiotics and prebiotics are said to help to keep it healthy – but do they work? You may have seen yoghurts or yoghurt drinks that contain probiotics on the supermarket shelves. These live cultures and yeasts are also available as supplements – and are frequently described as 'good' or 'gut-friendly' bacteria. The belief is that probiotics boost the number and variety of good bacteria in the colon, to help your digestive and possibly general health. Fermented vegetables such as kimchi (Korean pickled cabbage) and sauerkraut, miso and kefir (a fermented milk) are also naturally rich in probiotics and have become go-to health ingredients in recent years.

Do I need them?

Possibly. Probiotics may be useful for people who've been prescribed a course of antibiotics, which work by wiping out the bad (as well as some of the good) bacteria in your body as they fight infections. There is a fair bit of evidence that taking high doses of some probiotics can help prevent antibiotic-associated diarrhoea in children1 and reduce the risk of developing certain infections in adults.

Any issues?

Probiotic foods are generally fine for most of us and are a healthy addition to the diet, and people with a healthy immune system can usually take probiotic supplements without side effects. However, if you have any health issues that may mean your immune system is compromised, it's best to check with your GP before introducing a supplement to your diet. Also, as probiotics are classed as food rather than medicine, their effectiveness is less well established, as they don't have to undergo the same robust testing that medicines do3. Some small studies have shown that many of the bacteria in some probiotic products (mainly probiotic drinks) on the market are killed by our stomach acid and don't even make it to our intestines.

What are prebiotics then?

Prebiotics are non-digestible foods that stimulate the growth or activity of beneficial bacteria in the intestines. (The idea is that they provide the food that the probiotics need to thrive.) Examples are Jerusalem artichokes, leeks, onions, garlic, asparagus, bananas, legumes, honey, oats and lentils.

What are the benefits of these?
As well as the suggestion that they help 'good' bacteria to thrive, some studies have shown that prebiotics help our absorption of certain minerals[4] and can also be helpful in combating IBS[5]. Fibrous vegetables and grains will also help keep the bowels regular, so prebiotics are generally helpful for a healthy diet. That said, some people may experience bloating or flatulence if they suddenly add lots of these foods to their diet. Although there is still a need for more robust scientific testing on the influence of probiotics and prebiotics on our health[6] (especially in supplementary form), anecdotal evidence points to benefits for some.

However, there is no doubt that eating a varied diet, including a wide range of vegetables and fruit, is usually a very good idea.

LEAKY GUT DIET: WHAT TO EAT AND SAMPLE MEALS

The leaky gut diet refers to a way of eating that is intended to heal intestinal hyperpermeability, also known as leaky gut syndrome.Leaky gut syndrome is not an official medical diagnosis. It's a term used to explain a cluster of symptoms attributed to damage in the intestinal lining that allows larger particles to leak through. This can lead to digestive problems, nutrient deficiencies, autoimmune disorders, and other health issues. Leaky gut can be caused by gastrointestinal (GI) diseases, medications, or chemicals found in processed foods. Fortunately, research shows making dietary changes can help to heal a leaky gut.

How a Leaky Gut Might Affect You

Intestinal hyperpermeability interferes with digestion and can lead to body-wide inflammation. Under normal circumstances, the intestines absorb water and nutrients from what you eat and provide a protective barrier to keep bacteria and byproducts from getting into your bloodstream. This process is regulated by the size of the gaps (junctions) in the wall of your intestines. If the intestinal wall is damaged, cracks or holes can develop. These holes allow larger particles (partially digested food, bacteria, and toxins) to leak into the bloodstream. This can trigger an immune system reaction prompting systemic inflammation and illness. Leaky gut is often thought of as a digestive health issue, but it is also linked to a wide array of conditions. Symptoms that may be related to leaky gut include:

Abdominal bloating and gas

Acne

Allergies

Asthma

Autoimmune reactions

Chronic fatigue syndrome

Diarrhea

Fibromyalgia

Frequent infections

Headaches

Joint and muscle pain

Memory problems

Mood swings

Nonfatty liver disease

Obesity

Psoriasis

Type 1 diabetes

What Causes Leaky Gut Syndrome?

Leaky gut is more common in people with chronic GI conditions like celiac, inflammatory bowel disease (IBD), and irritable bowel syndrome (IBS). It may also be caused by common medications, like antibiotics, non-steroidal anti-inflammatory medicines (NSAIDs), and opioids.

Lifestyle factors—diet, alcohol, smoking, stress, and environmental toxins—also play a role.

Benefits of a Leaky Gut Diet

The leaky gut diet involves eating foods rich in certain nutrients while avoiding foods that irritate the digestive tract. Research shows following a leaky gut diet helps to:

Ease digestive symptoms

Relieve intestinal inflammation

Repair damage in the intestinal lining

Restore balance to the intestinal microbiome to improve gut health

The leaky gut diet may also relieve non-digestive symptoms related to intestinal hyperpermeability. Autoimmune diseases and inflammation, in particular, appear to benefit from the leaky gut diet.

Research shows nutritional compounds in the leaky gut diet help heal a leaky gut in the following ways:

Probiotics help to balance the intestinal microbiome and play other important roles in digestion and gut health.

Vitamins A and D help to repair the intestinal wall and regulate immune system responses.

Dietary fiber not only helps you stay regular, but it also stimulates the production of beneficial short-chain fatty acids and contains anti-inflammatory properties that protect the intestinal barrier.

Amino acids, like glutamine and arginine, help calm inflammation, regulate immune responses, and seal "leaky" gaps in the intestinal wall.

Polyphenols, plant compounds rich in antioxidants, combat oxidative stress that may contribute to intestinal permeability.

How Long to Follow a Leaky Gut Diet
The leaky gut diet may be used on a temporary or permanent basis. Some people only need to follow the diet temporarily to heal the intestinal lining and relieve short-term symptoms. If you're using a leaky gut diet to help treat

a chronic health condition, following the diet long-term can help prevent symptoms flares.

What to Eat on the Leaky Gut Diet

The leaky gut diet centers around whole, unprocessed foods with a focus on foods with nutrients that promote gut health. These include:

Fruits and veggies

Eggs

Chicken or turkey breast without the skin, lean cuts of pork

Fatty fish (salmon, tuna, herring)

Soups, bone broth

Cultured dairy products and dairy alternatives

Low-fat cheese

Tofu, tempeh, meat alternatives

Nuts and smooth nut butter

Sourdough bread, gluten-free grains, and whole grains

Flax, chia, and other seeds

Probiotic-rich fermented foods (yogurt, kombucha, kefir)

Water, coconut water, fruit juice without sugar, hot or iced tea

Fruits and Vegetables

Fruits and vegetables contain vitamins, minerals, and fiber that help to heal intestinal hyperpermeability and promote gut health. Plant-based sources of vitamin A include leafy greens like collard greens, kale, lettuce, spinach, and Swiss chard; yellow and orange fruits and vegetables like sweet potatoes, carrots, cantaloupe, and apricots; red peppers, tomatoes, broccoli, summer squash, and zucchini. Polyphenols resveratrol and quercetin are abundant in apples, blueberries, blackberries, citrus fruits, dark cherries, grapes, and onions. Mushrooms, the only plant-based source of vitamin D, contain other compounds that promote gut health. Look for chaga, king trumpet, maitake, lion's mane, shiitake, and turkey tail mushroom varieties, which have been shown in studies to reduce intestinal hyperpermeability. Fermented vegetables, like artichokes, kimchi, pickles, sauerkraut, and tempeh, are excellent sources of probiotics.

Grains

Grains can be beneficial or problematic, depending on the individual, and some grains are better for gut health than others. For example, wheat may trigger gastrointestinal symptoms in people who are sensitive to gluten. For people without gluten sensitivity, sourdough bread is recommended due to its probiotics. Whole grains, like brown rice and steel-cut oats, contain dietary fiber and other nutrients that support healthy digestion.1 However, large doses of fiber can also trigger GI symptoms. If you aren't already eating a lot of fiber, gradually add more to your diet.

Dairy

Yogurt and kefir containing live active probiotic cultures are considered the most beneficial foods for healing leaky gut. The only other dairy product recommended on the leaky gut diet is low-fat cheese. Dairy is generally problematic for people with GI disorders. Experts estimate two-thirds of adults have low levels of lactase, the enzyme that breaks down the sugar in dairy. Known as lactose intolerance, it causes bloating, diarrhea, and gas after consuming dairy. Products made from almond milk, cashew milk, coconut milk, and hemp milk are good dairy alternatives. However, these products may contain emulsifiers, like carrageenans, gums, or lecithins, that should be avoided on the leaky gut diet.

What Are the Best Probiotics for Leaky Gut Syndrome?
Studies show probiotics can help to reduce intestinal permeability and promote gut health in a number of other ways. Five probiotic strains beneficial for leaky gut syndrome include:

Lactobacillus (L.) acidophilus

L. plantarum

L. rhamnosus GG

Bifidobacterium (B.) animalis lactis BB-12

B. infantis

Protein

Animal proteins contain amino acids arginine and glutamine, which are the building blocks for repairing damaged intestinal walls. Egg yolks, liver, and fish are protein-rich sources of vitamin A, and fatty fish—trout, salmon, tuna, and mackerel—are excellent sources of vitamin D.914 Both vitamins are recommended for healing a leaky gut. Fermented soy products like tempeh and miso pack protein and probiotics that are beneficial for gut health. Tofu is also recommended on the leaky gut diet. Nuts, nut butters, and seeds are also good sources of protein, amino acids, and other nutrients known to support gut health. These foods are also high in fat, though, and can be difficult for some people with GI disorders to digest.

Beverages

Hydration is essential for digestive health, so be sure to drink plenty of water. Other drinks that can promote gut health include:

Ginger tea

Licorice root tea

Marshmallow root tea

Peppermint tea

Probiotic-rich fermented beverages like Kombucha and kefir

Tea from the Camellia Sinensis plant, which includes green, black, orange, white, or oolong teas

Herbs and Spices

Many herbs and spices contain polyphenols like berberine, catechin, curcumin, quercetin, and resveratrol that are beneficial for gut health. Spices recommended on the leaky gut diet include:

Basil

Celery seed

Cinnamon

Cloves

Cumin

Ginger

Lemon verbena

Marjoram

Oregano

Parsley

Peppermint

Rosemary

Sage

Thyme

Turmeric

Polyphenols Benefits and Foods to Eat

When to Eat
There is no set schedule for eating on the leaky gut diet. People with GI ailments often find eating smaller meals with snacks throughout the day helps to control their symptoms without going hungry.

Foods to Avoid with a Leaky Gut

The leaky gut diet eliminates excessive fats, sugars, additives, and ultra-processed foods. Research shows these foods contribute to intestinal hyperpermeability. The biggest offenders: sugar, salt, gluten, alcohol (and its metabolites), and emulsifiers. Foods to avoid on the leaky gut diet include:

Alcoholic beverages, including beer, wine, and liquor

Beans, legumes, corn, cruciferous vegetables

Bran, cereal or granola with nuts/fruit, dried fruit

Full-fat dairy products

Greasy, fatty, spicy, or fried foods

Lunchmeat, processed meat (hotdogs, sausage)

Pastries, cakes, cookies, candy, chocolate

Processed snack foods and desserts

Refined carbs and sugar

Sugar alcohols such as xylitol and sorbitol

Soda and energy drinks

Tough or fatty cuts of meat

Some people, particularly those with digestive health problems, may also want to stay off of foods that irritate their symptoms. This can include:

Caffeinated coffee and tea

Gluten, including bread, pasta, crackers

Brown, multigrain, or wild rice

Raw fruits and veggies with skin and seeds

What Are Emulsifiers?

Emulsifiers, food additives used to mix two substances that typically separate when combined, can contribute to leaky gut syndrome. They are found in many processed food products, including bread, baked goods, ice cream, margarine, and salad dressings. On the leaky gut diet, avoid products that contain the following emulsifiers:

Carboxymethylcellulose

Carrageenans

Guar gum

Lecithin

Locust bean gum

Maltodextrin

Polysorbate 80

Xantham gum

Who Should Follow the Leaky Gut Diet

Leaky gut syndrome is associated with GI diseases like IBD, IBS, and celiac, as well as non-GI conditions like autoimmune diseases, heart disease, obesity, and type 1 diabetes. The leaky gut diet is recommended for people who are experiencing gastrointestinal symptoms like bloating, constipation, diarrhea, and gas. People with allergies or a diagnosed autoimmune disease may also benefit from the eating plan. People who are experiencing unexplained symptoms like brain fog, fatigue, muscle and joint pain, or recurring infections may also find the leaky gut diet helpful.

Sample Menus
The leaky gut diet is centered around whole, unprocessed foods. This may require more meal prepping than you are used to. Aim to eat a variety of different foods throughout the week.

Breakfast

Breakfast ideas for the leaky gut diet include:

Egg-centered dishes like omelets, scrambled eggs with vegetables, or veggie frittatas. Stick to recipes that are dairy-free or allow low-fat cheese only. Add a side of fruit, roasted potatoes, or gluten-free toast

Greek yogurt mixed with fruit and nuts, like blueberries and sliced almonds or sliced bananas and walnuts.

Smoothies made with no-sugar-added yogurt or dairy-free milk. Add a mix of fruit, like berries or cherries, and leafy-green vegetables, like spinach or kale.

Steel-cut oats made with water or dairy-free milk. Add in fruit, nuts, or seeds and spices like cinnamon.

Tofu scramble made with crumbled firm or extra firm tofu seasoned with turmeric (to give it an egg-like appearance), leafy greens, and mushrooms.

Lunch

Ideas for lunch on the leaky gut diet include:

Bone-broth or miso soup and salad

Mixed leafy greens salad with hard-boiled eggs, grilled chicken breast, or salmon

Quinoa salad with vegetables and roasted turkey breast

Reheated leftovers from last night's dinner

Roasted beets with goat cheese and walnuts over baby greens

Sweet potatoes stuffed with ground turkey and vegetables

Steamed vegetables with fish or grilled chicken

Dinner

Dinner suggestions for the leaky gut diet include:

Beef and broccoli stir-fry with brown rice and kimchi

Grilled lemon chicken

Ground turkey and sautéed spinach and onions topped with mashed sweet potatoes

Pork chops with sauerkraut and sautéed apples or applesauce

Roasted chicken, vegetables, and potatoes

Roasted tempeh with carrots, Brussels sprouts, and quinoa

Steamed chicken and vegetables with brown rice

Zucchini ribbons topped with tomato sauce made with lean ground beef, mushrooms, onions, and peppersSnacks

If you get hungry between meals, try these healthy snack options on the leaky gut diet:

Crudité: Raw vegetables like celery sticks, carrot sticks, cucumbers, sliced bell peppers, broccoli, cauliflower, and asparagus spears

Fruit: Apples, berries, grapes, melon, pears, or other fruit

Guacamole: Use sliced red peppers or baby carrots instead of tortilla chips

Low-fat or nonfat cheese: Try part-skim string cheese or low-fat varieties of other cheeses, like cheddar, Colby, Gouda, or pepper-jack cheese

Nuts: Opt for dry-roasted unsalted nuts like almonds, cashews, pecans, pistachios, and walnuts

Seeds: Chia, flax, pumpkin, sesame, and sunflower flower seeds roasted without salt

Yogurt: No-sugar-added varieties that contain live active probioticsCooking Tips

The leaky gut diet relies on unprocessed foods, which means you may need to spend more time in the kitchen. One way to save time during the work week is to prep meals in advance on the weekend or double recipes to have leftovers. Portion meals into individual servings, store in the freezer, and reheat in the microwave when you are ready to eat.

Meals can also be made in a slow cooker (like a Crockpot), where the ingredients simmer together on a low setting over several hours, or in a pressure cooker (like an InstaPot), which uses high-pressure steam to shorten cooking time. Fermenting is another popular way to prepare food and boost its probiotic content, which may help regulate intestinal permeability. If you plan on eating in a restaurant or ordering takeout, look for gluten- and dairy-free dishes that are steamed, grilled, broiled, or roasted.

Avoid condiments, dressings, gravies, and sauces made with added sugar or thickened with wheat flour. Fried foods, which, in addition to being unhealthy, can be difficult to digest and should not be eaten on the leaky gut diet.

Tips for Special Health Needs

The leaky gut diet can be modified to accommodate special dietary needs and personal taste preferences. If you have food allergies or certain health conditions or are vegetarian, work with your healthcare provider or dietitian to ensure your nutritional needs are met. People with celiac disease need to avoid products with wheat or gluten. Avoid gluten-free products made with legume flours, such as chickpeas (garbanzo beans), fava beans, mung beans, navy beans, pinto beans, or white beans. Vegetarians will need to make sure they are eating enough plant-based proteins while also avoiding legumes. People with high cholesterol should limit their intake of saturated fat to less than 7% of total calories.17 People with hypertension need to limit their salt intake to 1,500 mg to 2,300 mg.18

Those with IBS or IBD may be advised to follow the low-FODMAP diet, which can be incorporated into the leaky gut diet. Many people with GI problems find it difficult to digest raw fruit and vegetables. Try boiling, grilling, roasting, microwaving, or steaming them instead. Fermented foods like kombucha, kimchi, and sauerkraut can cause digestive discomfort for some people. Start with small portions and gradually increase your intake of these foods or try yogurt or a probiotic supplement instead.

If your current diet does not contain a lot of fiber, add fiber-rich foods into your diet slowly to prevent GI upset. The Dietary Guidelines for Americans recommends 14 grams of fiber per 1,000 calories of food a day. If you eat 2,000 calories a day, slowly add more fiber to your diet until you reach 28 grams of fiber a day.

Side Effects of the Leaky Gut Diet
You might notice changes in your digestion any time you change how or what you eat. It's not unusual to have some temporary upset while your body adjusts. For example, if you alter the amount of fiber in your diet, you'll likely see a

direct effect on your bowel habits.   Usually, these changes will "level out" as your body gets used to your diet. However, if they do not or they get worse, you may need to reconsider the change. If you become constipated, drinking more water or adding a fiber supplement might be enough to correct it. Keeping a food and symptom journal can help to identify any foods that may be problematic to you.

BENEFITS OF A BLAND DIET FOR SYMPTOM MANAGEMENT

A bland diet consists of foods that are low in fiber and fat. Foods that are both low in fiber and fat are easier for your body to digest and are often referred to as low-residue or soft diets.1 Bland diets can be helpful during some medical conditions, as the foods are relatively non-irritating to the tissue in your mouth, throat, stomach, and intestines. Bland diets are not a dieting method for weight loss.

When Is a Bland Diet Useful?

Bland diets should only be considered for treating the symptoms of an underlying medical condition, and for as short a time as possible. Common reasons that your healthcare provider may recommend starting a bland diet can include:

Bacterial food poisoning: If possible, eat a bland diet and slowly return your diet to normal over one to two days as tolerated.

Gastroenteritis, also known as infectious diarrhea: Bland diets are usually better tolerated

Traveler's diarrhea: Bland diets may provide some comfort and nutrition while the common symptoms of an upset stomach may decrease your desire to eat.

Upset stomach

Nausea and vomiting of pregnancy (NVP), also known as hyperemesis gravidarum or morning sickness: Eating a bland diet in more frequent and smaller meals may help to relieve nausea.

Intermediate eating step after gastric surgery: A soft or bland diet is often used to advance your diet following surgery before you resume a regular diet.

Gastrointestinal bowel disease: A bland diet may be recommended to use during acute cases or flares of Crohn's, irritable bowel syndrome, inflammatory bowel disease, ulcerative colitis, or diverticulitis.

Bland diets are somewhat controversial in relation to diarrhea. Often, it's recommended to maintain a regular diet to ensure proper nutrition. However, due to the upset stomach and nausea that sometimes accompany diarrhea, a bland diet may be better tolerated.

Bland Diet vs. BRAT Diet

A BRAT diet is a diet that solely consists of bananas, rice, applesauce, and toast. While the BRAT diet is also considered a bland diet, it is more restrictive than the general bland diet. The intent behind the BRAT diet is to limit foods that are considered "binding," or provide bulk to your stool that makes it firmer. Bananas, which are high in potassium, are particularly helpful, as diarrhea will tend to cause you to lose potassium. While this may be a potentially useful diet for adults, this diet is no longer recommended for children.2 You may, however, discuss this option with your healthcare provider if your child cannot keep other foods down.

Otherwise, children are encouraged to maintain a normal diet. The BRAT diet should not be used long-term, as it is not sufficiently adequate in dietary requirements, and malnutrition will occur.

Foods to Eat

In general, foods that you eat on a bland diet do not have to taste bad or plain. There are many foods that can be eaten on a bland diet that you will likely find tasty to your palate. Listed below are categories of foods and some examples of foods that you can eat if you are on a bland diet:

Beverages: Herbal (decaffeinated) tea, water, juice, caffeine-free carbonated drinks, and sports drinks

Dairy: Milk (low-fat is preferred), yogurt, and cottage cheese

Desserts: Gelatin (flavored or plain), jam/jelly, honey, syrup, pound cake, sponge cake, and non-chocolate or peppermint custard, pudding, ice-cream, cookies, ice milk, and tapioca

Fats: Margarine, butter, mayonnaise, olive and canola oil, and mild salad dressings

Fruits: Bananas, applesauce, and fruit juices (may prefer to avoid citrus juice)

Grains: Cream of wheat, rice, and foods made with enriched flour, which include tortillas, white bread, English muffins, melba toast, rolls, pasta, and crackers

Proteins/Meats: Eggs, tofu, creamy peanut (or other nuts) butter, and well-cooked meat (with fat trimmed off), including chicken, fish, veal, lamb, and pork

Spices: Salt, cinnamon, thyme, allspice, paprika, ground spices in moderation, and prepared mustard

Vegetables: Potatoes and yams with skins that are baked, boiled, creamed, diced, or mashed

As you can see, there are many different types of foods that you can eat while maintaining a bland diet.

Foods to Avoid

Beverages: Alcohol, chocolate milk, coffee (both caffeinated and decaffeinated), and caffeinated teas or carbonated drinks

Dairy: Cocoa and chocolate drinks

Desserts: Desserts that contain chocolate, cocoa, or any spices that should be avoided

Fats: Strong salad dressings

Fruits: Raw fruits, citrus fruits, berries, and dried fruits

Grains: Fried foods, whole grains, and brown or wild rice

Proteins/Meats: Nuts, processed meat, spiced or seasoned meat, hot dogs, sausage, and fried meat or eggs

Spices: Pepper, chili powder, hot sauce, salsa, garlic, nutmeg, and other strong seasonings

Vegetables: Raw vegetables, peppers (mild or hot), and fried potatoesBland Diet Recipe Substitutes

As you can see from the lists above, a bland diet offers more variety than you may have originally assumed.

However, there are some limitations that may restrict you from eating some foods that you might usually enjoy.

While you can eat chicken while on a bland diet, you may find that you miss being able to add pepper to your meal. Instead, try using dried thyme on your chicken.

Nutmeg is a spice often included in many desserts. Try replacing nutmeg with cinnamon as an alternative spice for a tasty treat.

While you cannot duplicate the crunchy sensation of nuts in your recipes in a bland diet, you can often find a nut butter that you can use as a substitute to add flavor to your favorite dishes.

While you should avoid raw fruits, applesauce or other pureed fruits are acceptable to provide a fruit-filled treat.

If you are hooked on caffeine, you may find avoiding caffeinated beverages difficult. Try drinking herbal tea, coconut water, or sparkling water to curb your caffeine fix.

While fried eggs, meats, potatoes, or breads are to be avoided, try baking, broiling, or mashing these foods to replace fried substances in your meals.

Non-Gassy Foods: What to Eat to Reduce Gas and Bloating

To reduce bloating and farting, try including more non-gassy foods in your diet. Non-gassy foods include:

Red meat, poultry, or fish

Non-starchy vegetables, such as leafy greens and bell peppers

Fermented foods, such as kefir

Fruits, such as berries, in moderation

Rice, quinoa, or oats

Gluten-free bread or rice bread

Gassy foods, on the other hand, are foods that cause you to swallow air or that are less easy for your body to digest. Gassy foods include those that are high in sugar, starch, or fiber.1

Why Some Foods Cause Gas

As a general rule of thumb, gassy foods are those that contain certain types of carbohydrates (sugars and starch), soluble fiber (fiber that dissolves in water), or both. These substances are not fully absorbed in the small intestine and instead make their way down to the large intestine where they are broken down by gut bacteria.2 The product of this process is gas. You can avoid gas by eating less carbohydrates and soluble fiber. It is important to know that some gas is normal and that many gassy foods, like beans and broccoli, are good for you. Try to limit your diet to the non-gassy foods only when you absolutely must remain gas-free.

Animal Proteins

Protein sources that come from animals do not contain carbohydrates that are taken up by gut bacteria. So, choosing to eat animal proteins is a safe bet when you want to avoid gas or bloat. Glazes and gravy may contain added sugar, garlic, or onions, all of which can produce gas, so be sure to eat these items plain:

Beef

Chicken

Eggs

Fish

Turkey

If you choose not to eat animal products, there are plenty of other foods for you to enjoy.

LVegetables

Plenty of vegetables are low in carbohydrates and unlikely to cause gas. These are all good for you, so feel free to pile them onto your plate. You might even consider making a simple salad out of them and turning that into your big meal.

Bell peppers

Bok choy

Cucumber

Fennel

Greens, such as kale or spinach

Green beans

Lettuce

Spinach

Tomatoes

Zucchini

Fruits

A number of fruits are known for producing less gas. Still, it's a good idea to eat them in moderation. Your body can only absorb so many fruit-based carbohydrates at a time. The more fruit you eat—even of these less gassy options— the higher your chances are of having unwanted gas:

Blueberries

Cantaloupe

Clementine

Grapes

Honeydew

Kiwi

Pineapple

Raspberries

Strawberries

Fermented Foods

Bacteria found in fermented foods like yogurt have already taken care of the carbohydrates your gut would otherwise have to ferment.3 This frees your intestines from having to do all that work, which lowers the chance of gas. Bacteria from fermented foods are great for your gut's overall health. You really cannot go wrong with one of these choices:

Fermented vegetables

Kefir

Kombucha

Yogurt (without added sugars)

Grains

You may be surprised to learn that there are certain carbohydrates in wheat products that can lead to gas. The following choices are better options for the times when you just do not want to deal with gas:

Gluten-free bread

Rice bread

Oats

Rice, brown or white

Quinoa

Dairy Alternatives

Cow's milk contains lactose, a type of sugar that is harder for the body to digest, especially if you have lactose intolerance.bIf you regularly develop gas, bloating, diarrhea, vomiting, or upset stomach after eating dairy products, consider switching to a plant-based diary alternative, such as:

Almond milk

Coconut milk

Cashew milk

Oat milk

Rice milk

Hemp milk

Like beans, soy is a type of legume that can cause gas in some people. If you notice that soy products give you gas, take care to avoid them. While shopping for dairy alternatives, make sure to read ingredient lists carefully. Plant-based milks often contain added sugars, which can lead to gas.nDairy-free cheese, yogurt, butter, and ice cream alternatives are also available.

Snack Options

Along with the non-gassy vegetables and fruits, there are other good snack choices you can enjoy for a quick bite. Among those are nuts, but not every nut is reliable. Try to limit yourself to macadamia, pecans, and walnuts. You're also going to be pretty safe if you nibble on some cheese. For this, stick with cheddar, mozzarella, or Swiss.

Other Tips to Avoid Gas
Gas is a natural part of life, and you can't avoid it entirely. However, if you feel that your gas is excessive, there are some extra steps you can take.

Take Digestive Enzymes

Supplements containing digestive enzymes can help your body break down foods and absorb their nutrients better. This, in turn, should reduce gas. There are a few kinds of over-the-counter digestive enzyme supplements you can take depending on the type of food giving you gas:

Supplements containing the enzyme alpha galactosidase help your body break down the complex carbs in beans and vegetables that lead to gas.

Supplements containing the enzyme lactase help your body break down lactose—the gas-causing sugar in dairy products.

Supplements containing the enzyme lipase help your body break down fats in gassy foods so that your body can absorb them better.

If you are considering a digestive enzyme supplement, talk to your healthcare provider. Supplements are not FDA-regulated, so their exact ingredients and enzyme concentrations are not guaranteed. Your provider can recommend a digestive enzyme supplement that is most suitable for you.

Eat Slowly

Eating fast causes you to swallow more air, which can lead to gas. This problem is made worse by eating larger bites of food and failing to chew thoroughly; it is more difficult for the gastric juices in your stomach to degrade larger food particles. When you sit down for a meal, take your time and eat slowly. Take smaller bites, and chew your food well before swallowing. Make sure to drink plenty of fluids throughout your meal to help break down the food in your stomach.

Go for a Walk

Avoid lying down immediately after a meal and take yourself for a walk instead. One research study shows that walking for 10 to 15 minutes after a meal significantly reduces:7

Bloating

Belching

Flatulence

Abdominal pain and discomfort

The feeling of fullness

Furthermore, the study revealed that walking after a meal may even be as effective as medications for enhancing gastrointestinal motility (the movement of food through the digestive system).7

Try Process of Elimination

If you have been experiencing excessive gas, it helps to know what food is causing it so that you can remove it from your diet. The most efficient way to go about this is to use process of elimination. Start by removing one food from your diet at a time. If you suspect a certain food is giving you gas, stop eating it for a few days to see if your symptoms improve. If you are still having gas after removing the food, you will know that food isn't to blame. You can add it back into your diet and eliminate another food for a few days. You may find it helpful to keep track of the foods you remove and re-add by keeping a list. After you have removed a food and found that it was not the cause of your gas, write it down on your list under "non-gassy foods."

CONCLUSION

Foods that are higher in carbohydrates and soluble fiber are more likely to be fermented by gut bacteria and give you gas. You don't want to avoid these foods completely, though, since many foods with carbohydrates and soluble fiber are healthy. To avoid gas and bloating, choose animal proteins, leafy greens like spinach, fermented foods like kefir, and oats. Many fruits are good options too, but you should still eat them in moderation.

9 798869 742445